LOG BOOK  TO:

Name:

_____

DOB:

_____

Phone:

_____

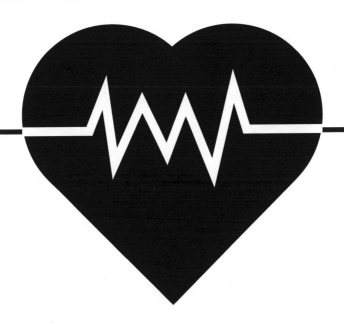

EMERGENCY CONTACTS

Name:

Phone:

Address:

Name:

Phone:

Address:

Notes:
_____
_____
_____
_____

MY DOCTOR'S CONTACT INFORMATION

Name:

Phone:

Address:

Notes:

_____

_____

_____

_____

_____

_____

_____

_____

_____

_____

_____

_____

_____

MY PHARMACIST'S CONTACT INFORMATION

Name:

Phone:

Address:

Notes:

_____

_____

_____

_____

_____

_____

_____

_____

_____

_____

Weekly Blood Sugar Log

Week: _____ to _____

	Time	Before	After	Notes
MONDAY	Breakfast			
	Lunch			
	Dinner			
	Bedtime			
TUESDAY	Breakfast			
	Lunch			
	Dinner			
	Bedtime			
WEDNESDAY	Breakfast			
	Lunch			
	Dinner			
	Bedtime			
THURSDAY	Breakfast			
	Lunch			
	Dinner			
	Bedtime			
FRIDAY	Breakfast			
	Lunch			
	Dinner			
	Bedtime			
SATURDAY	Breakfast			
	Lunch			
	Dinner			
	Bedtime			
SUNDAY	Breakfast			
	Lunch			
	Dinner			
	Bedtime			

Weekly Blood Sugar Log

Week: _____ to _____

	Time	Before	After	Notes
MONDAY	Breakfast			
	Lunch			
	Dinner			
	Bedtime			
TUESDAY	Breakfast			
	Lunch			
	Dinner			
	Bedtime			
WEDNESDAY	Breakfast			
	Lunch			
	Dinner			
	Bedtime			
THURSDAY	Breakfast			
	Lunch			
	Dinner			
	Bedtime			
FRIDAY	Breakfast			
	Lunch			
	Dinner			
	Bedtime			
SATURDAY	Breakfast			
	Lunch			
	Dinner			
	Bedtime			
SUNDAY	Breakfast			
	Lunch			
	Dinner			
	Bedtime			

Weekly Blood Sugar Log

Week: _____ to _____

	Time	Before	After	Notes
MONDAY	Breakfast			
	Lunch			
	Dinner			
	Bedtime			
TUESDAY	Breakfast			
	Lunch			
	Dinner			
	Bedtime			
WEDNESDAY	Breakfast			
	Lunch			
	Dinner			
	Bedtime			
THURSDAY	Breakfast			
	Lunch			
	Dinner			
	Bedtime			
FRIDAY	Breakfast			
	Lunch			
	Dinner			
	Bedtime			
SATURDAY	Breakfast			
	Lunch			
	Dinner			
	Bedtime			
SUNDAY	Breakfast			
	Lunch			
	Dinner			
	Bedtime			

Weekly Blood Sugar Log

Week: _____ to _____

	Time	Before	After	Notes
MONDAY	Breakfast			
	Lunch			
	Dinner			
	Bedtime			
TUESDAY	Breakfast			
	Lunch			
	Dinner			
	Bedtime			
WEDNESDAY	Breakfast			
	Lunch			
	Dinner			
	Bedtime			
THURSDAY	Breakfast			
	Lunch			
	Dinner			
	Bedtime			
FRIDAY	Breakfast			
	Lunch			
	Dinner			
	Bedtime			
SATURDAY	Breakfast			
	Lunch			
	Dinner			
	Bedtime			
SUNDAY	Breakfast			
	Lunch			
	Dinner			
	Bedtime			

Weekly Blood Sugar Log

Week: _____ to _____

	Time	Before	After	Notes
MONDAY	Breakfast			
	Lunch			
	Dinner			
	Bedtime			
TUESDAY	Breakfast			
	Lunch			
	Dinner			
	Bedtime			
WEDNESDAY	Breakfast			
	Lunch			
	Dinner			
	Bedtime			
THURSDAY	Breakfast			
	Lunch			
	Dinner			
	Bedtime			
FRIDAY	Breakfast			
	Lunch			
	Dinner			
	Bedtime			
SATURDAY	Breakfast			
	Lunch			
	Dinner			
	Bedtime			
SUNDAY	Breakfast			
	Lunch			
	Dinner			
	Bedtime			

Weekly Blood Sugar Log

Week: _____ to _____

	Time	Before	After	Notes
MONDAY	Breakfast			
	Lunch			
	Dinner			
	Bedtime			
TUESDAY	Breakfast			
	Lunch			
	Dinner			
	Bedtime			
WEDNESDAY	Breakfast			
	Lunch			
	Dinner			
	Bedtime			
THURSDAY	Breakfast			
	Lunch			
	Dinner			
	Bedtime			
FRIDAY	Breakfast			
	Lunch			
	Dinner			
	Bedtime			
SATURDAY	Breakfast			
	Lunch			
	Dinner			
	Bedtime			
SUNDAY	Breakfast			
	Lunch			
	Dinner			
	Bedtime			

Weekly Blood Sugar Log

Week: _____ to _____

	Time	Before	After	Notes
MONDAY	Breakfast			
	Lunch			
	Dinner			
	Bedtime			
TUESDAY	Breakfast			
	Lunch			
	Dinner			
	Bedtime			
WEDNESDAY	Breakfast			
	Lunch			
	Dinner			
	Bedtime			
THURSDAY	Breakfast			
	Lunch			
	Dinner			
	Bedtime			
FRIDAY	Breakfast			
	Lunch			
	Dinner			
	Bedtime			
SATURDAY	Breakfast			
	Lunch			
	Dinner			
	Bedtime			
SUNDAY	Breakfast			
	Lunch			
	Dinner			
	Bedtime			

Weekly Blood Sugar Log

Week: _____ to _____

	Time	Before	After	Notes
MONDAY	Breakfast			
	Lunch			
	Dinner			
	Bedtime			
TUESDAY	Breakfast			
	Lunch			
	Dinner			
	Bedtime			
WEDNESDAY	Breakfast			
	Lunch			
	Dinner			
	Bedtime			
THURSDAY	Breakfast			
	Lunch			
	Dinner			
	Bedtime			
FRIDAY	Breakfast			
	Lunch			
	Dinner			
	Bedtime			
SATURDAY	Breakfast			
	Lunch			
	Dinner			
	Bedtime			
SUNDAY	Breakfast			
	Lunch			
	Dinner			
	Bedtime			

Weekly Blood Sugar Log

Week: _____ to _____

	Time	Before	After	Notes
MONDAY	Breakfast			
	Lunch			
	Dinner			
	Bedtime			
TUESDAY	Breakfast			
	Lunch			
	Dinner			
	Bedtime			
WEDNESDAY	Breakfast			
	Lunch			
	Dinner			
	Bedtime			
THURSDAY	Breakfast			
	Lunch			
	Dinner			
	Bedtime			
FRIDAY	Breakfast			
	Lunch			
	Dinner			
	Bedtime			
SATURDAY	Breakfast			
	Lunch			
	Dinner			
	Bedtime			
SUNDAY	Breakfast			
	Lunch			
	Dinner			
	Bedtime			

Weekly Blood Sugar Log

Week: _____ to _____

	Time	Before	After	Notes
MONDAY	Breakfast			
	Lunch			
	Dinner			
	Bedtime			
TUESDAY	Breakfast			
	Lunch			
	Dinner			
	Bedtime			
WEDNESDAY	Breakfast			
	Lunch			
	Dinner			
	Bedtime			
THURSDAY	Breakfast			
	Lunch			
	Dinner			
	Bedtime			
FRIDAY	Breakfast			
	Lunch			
	Dinner			
	Bedtime			
SATURDAY	Breakfast			
	Lunch			
	Dinner			
	Bedtime			
SUNDAY	Breakfast			
	Lunch			
	Dinner			
	Bedtime			

Weekly Blood Sugar Log

Week: _____ to _____

	Time	Before	After	Notes
MONDAY	Breakfast			
	Lunch			
	Dinner			
	Bedtime			
TUESDAY	Breakfast			
	Lunch			
	Dinner			
	Bedtime			
WEDNESDAY	Breakfast			
	Lunch			
	Dinner			
	Bedtime			
THURSDAY	Breakfast			
	Lunch			
	Dinner			
	Bedtime			
FRIDAY	Breakfast			
	Lunch			
	Dinner			
	Bedtime			
SATURDAY	Breakfast			
	Lunch			
	Dinner			
	Bedtime			
SUNDAY	Breakfast			
	Lunch			
	Dinner			
	Bedtime			

Weekly Blood Sugar Log

Week: _____ to _____

	Time	Before	After	Notes
MONDAY	Breakfast			
	Lunch			
	Dinner			
	Bedtime			
TUESDAY	Breakfast			
	Lunch			
	Dinner			
	Bedtime			
WEDNESDAY	Breakfast			
	Lunch			
	Dinner			
	Bedtime			
THURSDAY	Breakfast			
	Lunch			
	Dinner			
	Bedtime			
FRIDAY	Breakfast			
	Lunch			
	Dinner			
	Bedtime			
SATURDAY	Breakfast			
	Lunch			
	Dinner			
	Bedtime			
SUNDAY	Breakfast			
	Lunch			
	Dinner			
	Bedtime			

Weekly Blood Sugar Log

Week: _____ to _____

	Time	Before	After	Notes
MONDAY	Breakfast			
	Lunch			
	Dinner			
	Bedtime			
TUESDAY	Breakfast			
	Lunch			
	Dinner			
	Bedtime			
WEDNESDAY	Breakfast			
	Lunch			
	Dinner			
	Bedtime			
THURSDAY	Breakfast			
	Lunch			
	Dinner			
	Bedtime			
FRIDAY	Breakfast			
	Lunch			
	Dinner			
	Bedtime			
SATURDAY	Breakfast			
	Lunch			
	Dinner			
	Bedtime			
SUNDAY	Breakfast			
	Lunch			
	Dinner			
	Bedtime			

Weekly Blood Sugar Log

Week: _____ to _____

	Time	Before	After	Notes
MONDAY	Breakfast			
	Lunch			
	Dinner			
	Bedtime			
TUESDAY	Breakfast			
	Lunch			
	Dinner			
	Bedtime			
WEDNESDAY	Breakfast			
	Lunch			
	Dinner			
	Bedtime			
THURSDAY	Breakfast			
	Lunch			
	Dinner			
	Bedtime			
FRIDAY	Breakfast			
	Lunch			
	Dinner			
	Bedtime			
SATURDAY	Breakfast			
	Lunch			
	Dinner			
	Bedtime			
SUNDAY	Breakfast			
	Lunch			
	Dinner			
	Bedtime			

Weekly Blood Sugar Log

Week: _____ to _____

	Time	Before	After	Notes
MONDAY	Breakfast			
	Lunch			
	Dinner			
	Bedtime			
TUESDAY	Breakfast			
	Lunch			
	Dinner			
	Bedtime			
WEDNESDAY	Breakfast			
	Lunch			
	Dinner			
	Bedtime			
THURSDAY	Breakfast			
	Lunch			
	Dinner			
	Bedtime			
FRIDAY	Breakfast			
	Lunch			
	Dinner			
	Bedtime			
SATURDAY	Breakfast			
	Lunch			
	Dinner			
	Bedtime			
SUNDAY	Breakfast			
	Lunch			
	Dinner			
	Bedtime			

Weekly Blood Sugar Log

Week: _____ to _____

	Time	Before	After	Notes
MONDAY	Breakfast			
	Lunch			
	Dinner			
	Bedtime			
TUESDAY	Breakfast			
	Lunch			
	Dinner			
	Bedtime			
WEDNESDAY	Breakfast			
	Lunch			
	Dinner			
	Bedtime			
THURSDAY	Breakfast			
	Lunch			
	Dinner			
	Bedtime			
FRIDAY	Breakfast			
	Lunch			
	Dinner			
	Bedtime			
SATURDAY	Breakfast			
	Lunch			
	Dinner			
	Bedtime			
SUNDAY	Breakfast			
	Lunch			
	Dinner			
	Bedtime			

Weekly Blood Sugar Log

Week: _____ to _____

	Time	Before	After	Notes
MONDAY	Breakfast			
	Lunch			
	Dinner			
	Bedtime			
TUESDAY	Breakfast			
	Lunch			
	Dinner			
	Bedtime			
WEDNESDAY	Breakfast			
	Lunch			
	Dinner			
	Bedtime			
THURSDAY	Breakfast			
	Lunch			
	Dinner			
	Bedtime			
FRIDAY	Breakfast			
	Lunch			
	Dinner			
	Bedtime			
SATURDAY	Breakfast			
	Lunch			
	Dinner			
	Bedtime			
SUNDAY	Breakfast			
	Lunch			
	Dinner			
	Bedtime			

Weekly Blood Sugar Log

Week: _____ to _____

	Time	Before	After	Notes
MONDAY	Breakfast			
	Lunch			
	Dinner			
	Bedtime			
TUESDAY	Breakfast			
	Lunch			
	Dinner			
	Bedtime			
WEDNESDAY	Breakfast			
	Lunch			
	Dinner			
	Bedtime			
THURSDAY	Breakfast			
	Lunch			
	Dinner			
	Bedtime			
FRIDAY	Breakfast			
	Lunch			
	Dinner			
	Bedtime			
SATURDAY	Breakfast			
	Lunch			
	Dinner			
	Bedtime			
SUNDAY	Breakfast			
	Lunch			
	Dinner			
	Bedtime			

Weekly Blood Sugar Log

Week: _____ to _____

	Time	Before	After	Notes
MONDAY	Breakfast			
	Lunch			
	Dinner			
	Bedtime			
TUESDAY	Breakfast			
	Lunch			
	Dinner			
	Bedtime			
WEDNESDAY	Breakfast			
	Lunch			
	Dinner			
	Bedtime			
THURSDAY	Breakfast			
	Lunch			
	Dinner			
	Bedtime			
FRIDAY	Breakfast			
	Lunch			
	Dinner			
	Bedtime			
SATURDAY	Breakfast			
	Lunch			
	Dinner			
	Bedtime			
SUNDAY	Breakfast			
	Lunch			
	Dinner			
	Bedtime			

Weekly Blood Sugar Log

Week: _____ to _____

	Time	Before	After	Notes
MONDAY	Breakfast			
	Lunch			
	Dinner			
	Bedtime			
TUESDAY	Breakfast			
	Lunch			
	Dinner			
	Bedtime			
WEDNESDAY	Breakfast			
	Lunch			
	Dinner			
	Bedtime			
THURSDAY	Breakfast			
	Lunch			
	Dinner			
	Bedtime			
FRIDAY	Breakfast			
	Lunch			
	Dinner			
	Bedtime			
SATURDAY	Breakfast			
	Lunch			
	Dinner			
	Bedtime			
SUNDAY	Breakfast			
	Lunch			
	Dinner			
	Bedtime			

Weekly Blood Sugar Log

Week: _____ to _____

	Time	Before	After	Notes
MONDAY	Breakfast			
	Lunch			
	Dinner			
	Bedtime			
TUESDAY	Breakfast			
	Lunch			
	Dinner			
	Bedtime			
WEDNESDAY	Breakfast			
	Lunch			
	Dinner			
	Bedtime			
THURSDAY	Breakfast			
	Lunch			
	Dinner			
	Bedtime			
FRIDAY	Breakfast			
	Lunch			
	Dinner			
	Bedtime			
SATURDAY	Breakfast			
	Lunch			
	Dinner			
	Bedtime			
SUNDAY	Breakfast			
	Lunch			
	Dinner			
	Bedtime			

Weekly Blood Sugar Log

Week: _____ to _____

	Time	Before	After	Notes
MONDAY	Breakfast			
	Lunch			
	Dinner			
	Bedtime			
TUESDAY	Breakfast			
	Lunch			
	Dinner			
	Bedtime			
WEDNESDAY	Breakfast			
	Lunch			
	Dinner			
	Bedtime			
THURSDAY	Breakfast			
	Lunch			
	Dinner			
	Bedtime			
FRIDAY	Breakfast			
	Lunch			
	Dinner			
	Bedtime			
SATURDAY	Breakfast			
	Lunch			
	Dinner			
	Bedtime			
SUNDAY	Breakfast			
	Lunch			
	Dinner			
	Bedtime			

Weekly Blood Sugar Log

Week: _____ to _____

	Time	Before	After	Notes
MONDAY	Breakfast			
	Lunch			
	Dinner			
	Bedtime			
TUESDAY	Breakfast			
	Lunch			
	Dinner			
	Bedtime			
WEDNESDAY	Breakfast			
	Lunch			
	Dinner			
	Bedtime			
THURSDAY	Breakfast			
	Lunch			
	Dinner			
	Bedtime			
FRIDAY	Breakfast			
	Lunch			
	Dinner			
	Bedtime			
SATURDAY	Breakfast			
	Lunch			
	Dinner			
	Bedtime			
SUNDAY	Breakfast			
	Lunch			
	Dinner			
	Bedtime			

Weekly Blood Sugar Log

Week: _____ to _____

	Time	Before	After	Notes
MONDAY	Breakfast			
	Lunch			
	Dinner			
	Bedtime			
TUESDAY	Breakfast			
	Lunch			
	Dinner			
	Bedtime			
WEDNESDAY	Breakfast			
	Lunch			
	Dinner			
	Bedtime			
THURSDAY	Breakfast			
	Lunch			
	Dinner			
	Bedtime			
FRIDAY	Breakfast			
	Lunch			
	Dinner			
	Bedtime			
SATURDAY	Breakfast			
	Lunch			
	Dinner			
	Bedtime			
SUNDAY	Breakfast			
	Lunch			
	Dinner			
	Bedtime			

Weekly Blood Sugar Log

Week: _____ to _____

	Time	Before	After	Notes
MONDAY	Breakfast			
	Lunch			
	Dinner			
	Bedtime			
TUESDAY	Breakfast			
	Lunch			
	Dinner			
	Bedtime			
WEDNESDAY	Breakfast			
	Lunch			
	Dinner			
	Bedtime			
THURSDAY	Breakfast			
	Lunch			
	Dinner			
	Bedtime			
FRIDAY	Breakfast			
	Lunch			
	Dinner			
	Bedtime			
SATURDAY	Breakfast			
	Lunch			
	Dinner			
	Bedtime			
SUNDAY	Breakfast			
	Lunch			
	Dinner			
	Bedtime			

Weekly Blood Sugar Log

Week: _____ to _____

	Time	Before	After	Notes
MONDAY	Breakfast			
	Lunch			
	Dinner			
	Bedtime			
TUESDAY	Breakfast			
	Lunch			
	Dinner			
	Bedtime			
WEDNESDAY	Breakfast			
	Lunch			
	Dinner			
	Bedtime			
THURSDAY	Breakfast			
	Lunch			
	Dinner			
	Bedtime			
FRIDAY	Breakfast			
	Lunch			
	Dinner			
	Bedtime			
SATURDAY	Breakfast			
	Lunch			
	Dinner			
	Bedtime			
SUNDAY	Breakfast			
	Lunch			
	Dinner			
	Bedtime			

Weekly Blood Sugar Log

Week: _____ to _____

	Time	Before	After	Notes
MONDAY	Breakfast			
	Lunch			
	Dinner			
	Bedtime			
TUESDAY	Breakfast			
	Lunch			
	Dinner			
	Bedtime			
WEDNESDAY	Breakfast			
	Lunch			
	Dinner			
	Bedtime			
THURSDAY	Breakfast			
	Lunch			
	Dinner			
	Bedtime			
FRIDAY	Breakfast			
	Lunch			
	Dinner			
	Bedtime			
SATURDAY	Breakfast			
	Lunch			
	Dinner			
	Bedtime			
SUNDAY	Breakfast			
	Lunch			
	Dinner			
	Bedtime			

Weekly Blood Sugar Log

Week: _____ to _____

	Time	Before	After	Notes
MONDAY	Breakfast			
	Lunch			
	Dinner			
	Bedtime			
TUESDAY	Breakfast			
	Lunch			
	Dinner			
	Bedtime			
WEDNESDAY	Breakfast			
	Lunch			
	Dinner			
	Bedtime			
THURSDAY	Breakfast			
	Lunch			
	Dinner			
	Bedtime			
FRIDAY	Breakfast			
	Lunch			
	Dinner			
	Bedtime			
SATURDAY	Breakfast			
	Lunch			
	Dinner			
	Bedtime			
SUNDAY	Breakfast			
	Lunch			
	Dinner			
	Bedtime			

Weekly Blood Sugar Log

Week: _____ to _____

	Time	Before	After	Notes
MONDAY	Breakfast			
	Lunch			
	Dinner			
	Bedtime			
TUESDAY	Breakfast			
	Lunch			
	Dinner			
	Bedtime			
WEDNESDAY	Breakfast			
	Lunch			
	Dinner			
	Bedtime			
THURSDAY	Breakfast			
	Lunch			
	Dinner			
	Bedtime			
FRIDAY	Breakfast			
	Lunch			
	Dinner			
	Bedtime			
SATURDAY	Breakfast			
	Lunch			
	Dinner			
	Bedtime			
SUNDAY	Breakfast			
	Lunch			
	Dinner			
	Bedtime			

Weekly Blood Sugar Log

Week: _____ to _____

	Time	Before	After	Notes
MONDAY	Breakfast			
	Lunch			
	Dinner			
	Bedtime			
TUESDAY	Breakfast			
	Lunch			
	Dinner			
	Bedtime			
WEDNESDAY	Breakfast			
	Lunch			
	Dinner			
	Bedtime			
THURSDAY	Breakfast			
	Lunch			
	Dinner			
	Bedtime			
FRIDAY	Breakfast			
	Lunch			
	Dinner			
	Bedtime			
SATURDAY	Breakfast			
	Lunch			
	Dinner			
	Bedtime			
SUNDAY	Breakfast			
	Lunch			
	Dinner			
	Bedtime			

Weekly Blood Sugar Log

Week: _____ to _____

	Time	Before	After	Notes
MONDAY	Breakfast			
	Lunch			
	Dinner			
	Bedtime			
TUESDAY	Breakfast			
	Lunch			
	Dinner			
	Bedtime			
WEDNESDAY	Breakfast			
	Lunch			
	Dinner			
	Bedtime			
THURSDAY	Breakfast			
	Lunch			
	Dinner			
	Bedtime			
FRIDAY	Breakfast			
	Lunch			
	Dinner			
	Bedtime			
SATURDAY	Breakfast			
	Lunch			
	Dinner			
	Bedtime			
SUNDAY	Breakfast			
	Lunch			
	Dinner			
	Bedtime			

Weekly Blood Sugar Log

Week: _____ to _____

	Time	Before	After	Notes
MONDAY	Breakfast			
	Lunch			
	Dinner			
	Bedtime			
TUESDAY	Breakfast			
	Lunch			
	Dinner			
	Bedtime			
WEDNESDAY	Breakfast			
	Lunch			
	Dinner			
	Bedtime			
THURSDAY	Breakfast			
	Lunch			
	Dinner			
	Bedtime			
FRIDAY	Breakfast			
	Lunch			
	Dinner			
	Bedtime			
SATURDAY	Breakfast			
	Lunch			
	Dinner			
	Bedtime			
SUNDAY	Breakfast			
	Lunch			
	Dinner			
	Bedtime			

Weekly Blood Sugar Log

Week: _____ to _____

	Time	Before	After	Notes
MONDAY	Breakfast			
	Lunch			
	Dinner			
	Bedtime			
TUESDAY	Breakfast			
	Lunch			
	Dinner			
	Bedtime			
WEDNESDAY	Breakfast			
	Lunch			
	Dinner			
	Bedtime			
THURSDAY	Breakfast			
	Lunch			
	Dinner			
	Bedtime			
FRIDAY	Breakfast			
	Lunch			
	Dinner			
	Bedtime			
SATURDAY	Breakfast			
	Lunch			
	Dinner			
	Bedtime			
SUNDAY	Breakfast			
	Lunch			
	Dinner			
	Bedtime			

Weekly Blood Sugar Log

Week: _____ to _____

	Time	Before	After	Notes
MONDAY	Breakfast			
	Lunch			
	Dinner			
	Bedtime			
TUESDAY	Breakfast			
	Lunch			
	Dinner			
	Bedtime			
WEDNESDAY	Breakfast			
	Lunch			
	Dinner			
	Bedtime			
THURSDAY	Breakfast			
	Lunch			
	Dinner			
	Bedtime			
FRIDAY	Breakfast			
	Lunch			
	Dinner			
	Bedtime			
SATURDAY	Breakfast			
	Lunch			
	Dinner			
	Bedtime			
SUNDAY	Breakfast			
	Lunch			
	Dinner			
	Bedtime			

Weekly Blood Sugar Log

Week: _____ to _____

	Time	Before	After	Notes
MONDAY	Breakfast			
	Lunch			
	Dinner			
	Bedtime			
TUESDAY	Breakfast			
	Lunch			
	Dinner			
	Bedtime			
WEDNESDAY	Breakfast			
	Lunch			
	Dinner			
	Bedtime			
THURSDAY	Breakfast			
	Lunch			
	Dinner			
	Bedtime			
FRIDAY	Breakfast			
	Lunch			
	Dinner			
	Bedtime			
SATURDAY	Breakfast			
	Lunch			
	Dinner			
	Bedtime			
SUNDAY	Breakfast			
	Lunch			
	Dinner			
	Bedtime			

Weekly Blood Sugar Log

Week: _____ to _____

	Time	Before	After	Notes
MONDAY	Breakfast			
	Lunch			
	Dinner			
	Bedtime			
TUESDAY	Breakfast			
	Lunch			
	Dinner			
	Bedtime			
WEDNESDAY	Breakfast			
	Lunch			
	Dinner			
	Bedtime			
THURSDAY	Breakfast			
	Lunch			
	Dinner			
	Bedtime			
FRIDAY	Breakfast			
	Lunch			
	Dinner			
	Bedtime			
SATURDAY	Breakfast			
	Lunch			
	Dinner			
	Bedtime			
SUNDAY	Breakfast			
	Lunch			
	Dinner			
	Bedtime			

Weekly Blood Sugar Log

Week: _____ to _____

	Time	Before	After	Notes
MONDAY	Breakfast			
	Lunch			
	Dinner			
	Bedtime			
TUESDAY	Breakfast			
	Lunch			
	Dinner			
	Bedtime			
WEDNESDAY	Breakfast			
	Lunch			
	Dinner			
	Bedtime			
THURSDAY	Breakfast			
	Lunch			
	Dinner			
	Bedtime			
FRIDAY	Breakfast			
	Lunch			
	Dinner			
	Bedtime			
SATURDAY	Breakfast			
	Lunch			
	Dinner			
	Bedtime			
SUNDAY	Breakfast			
	Lunch			
	Dinner			
	Bedtime			

Weekly Blood Sugar Log

Week: _____ to _____

	Time	Before	After	Notes
MONDAY	Breakfast			
	Lunch			
	Dinner			
	Bedtime			
TUESDAY	Breakfast			
	Lunch			
	Dinner			
	Bedtime			
WEDNESDAY	Breakfast			
	Lunch			
	Dinner			
	Bedtime			
THURSDAY	Breakfast			
	Lunch			
	Dinner			
	Bedtime			
FRIDAY	Breakfast			
	Lunch			
	Dinner			
	Bedtime			
SATURDAY	Breakfast			
	Lunch			
	Dinner			
	Bedtime			
SUNDAY	Breakfast			
	Lunch			
	Dinner			
	Bedtime			

Weekly Blood Sugar Log

Week: _____ to _____

	Time	Before	After	Notes
MONDAY	Breakfast			
	Lunch			
	Dinner			
	Bedtime			
TUESDAY	Breakfast			
	Lunch			
	Dinner			
	Bedtime			
WEDNESDAY	Breakfast			
	Lunch			
	Dinner			
	Bedtime			
THURSDAY	Breakfast			
	Lunch			
	Dinner			
	Bedtime			
FRIDAY	Breakfast			
	Lunch			
	Dinner			
	Bedtime			
SATURDAY	Breakfast			
	Lunch			
	Dinner			
	Bedtime			
SUNDAY	Breakfast			
	Lunch			
	Dinner			
	Bedtime			

Weekly Blood Sugar Log

Week: _____ to _____

	Time	Before	After	Notes
MONDAY	Breakfast			
	Lunch			
	Dinner			
	Bedtime			
TUESDAY	Breakfast			
	Lunch			
	Dinner			
	Bedtime			
WEDNESDAY	Breakfast			
	Lunch			
	Dinner			
	Bedtime			
THURSDAY	Breakfast			
	Lunch			
	Dinner			
	Bedtime			
FRIDAY	Breakfast			
	Lunch			
	Dinner			
	Bedtime			
SATURDAY	Breakfast			
	Lunch			
	Dinner			
	Bedtime			
SUNDAY	Breakfast			
	Lunch			
	Dinner			
	Bedtime			

Weekly Blood Sugar Log

Week: _____ to _____

	Time	Before	After	Notes
MONDAY	Breakfast			
	Lunch			
	Dinner			
	Bedtime			
TUESDAY	Breakfast			
	Lunch			
	Dinner			
	Bedtime			
WEDNESDAY	Breakfast			
	Lunch			
	Dinner			
	Bedtime			
THURSDAY	Breakfast			
	Lunch			
	Dinner			
	Bedtime			
FRIDAY	Breakfast			
	Lunch			
	Dinner			
	Bedtime			
SATURDAY	Breakfast			
	Lunch			
	Dinner			
	Bedtime			
SUNDAY	Breakfast			
	Lunch			
	Dinner			
	Bedtime			

Weekly Blood Sugar Log

Week: _____ to _____

	Time	Before	After	Notes
MONDAY	Breakfast			
	Lunch			
	Dinner			
	Bedtime			
TUESDAY	Breakfast			
	Lunch			
	Dinner			
	Bedtime			
WEDNESDAY	Breakfast			
	Lunch			
	Dinner			
	Bedtime			
THURSDAY	Breakfast			
	Lunch			
	Dinner			
	Bedtime			
FRIDAY	Breakfast			
	Lunch			
	Dinner			
	Bedtime			
SATURDAY	Breakfast			
	Lunch			
	Dinner			
	Bedtime			
SUNDAY	Breakfast			
	Lunch			
	Dinner			
	Bedtime			

Weekly Blood Sugar Log

Week: _____ to _____

	Time	Before	After	Notes
MONDAY	Breakfast			
	Lunch			
	Dinner			
	Bedtime			
TUESDAY	Breakfast			
	Lunch			
	Dinner			
	Bedtime			
WEDNESDAY	Breakfast			
	Lunch			
	Dinner			
	Bedtime			
THURSDAY	Breakfast			
	Lunch			
	Dinner			
	Bedtime			
FRIDAY	Breakfast			
	Lunch			
	Dinner			
	Bedtime			
SATURDAY	Breakfast			
	Lunch			
	Dinner			
	Bedtime			
SUNDAY	Breakfast			
	Lunch			
	Dinner			
	Bedtime			

Weekly Blood Sugar Log

Week: _____ to _____

	Time	Before	After	Notes
MONDAY	Breakfast			
	Lunch			
	Dinner			
	Bedtime			
TUESDAY	Breakfast			
	Lunch			
	Dinner			
	Bedtime			
WEDNESDAY	Breakfast			
	Lunch			
	Dinner			
	Bedtime			
THURSDAY	Breakfast			
	Lunch			
	Dinner			
	Bedtime			
FRIDAY	Breakfast			
	Lunch			
	Dinner			
	Bedtime			
SATURDAY	Breakfast			
	Lunch			
	Dinner			
	Bedtime			
SUNDAY	Breakfast			
	Lunch			
	Dinner			
	Bedtime			

Weekly Blood Sugar Log

Week: _____ to _____

	Time	Before	After	Notes
MONDAY	Breakfast			
	Lunch			
	Dinner			
	Bedtime			
TUESDAY	Breakfast			
	Lunch			
	Dinner			
	Bedtime			
WEDNESDAY	Breakfast			
	Lunch			
	Dinner			
	Bedtime			
THURSDAY	Breakfast			
	Lunch			
	Dinner			
	Bedtime			
FRIDAY	Breakfast			
	Lunch			
	Dinner			
	Bedtime			
SATURDAY	Breakfast			
	Lunch			
	Dinner			
	Bedtime			
SUNDAY	Breakfast			
	Lunch			
	Dinner			
	Bedtime			

Weekly Blood Sugar Log

Week: _____ to _____

	Time	Before	After	Notes
MONDAY	Breakfast			
	Lunch			
	Dinner			
	Bedtime			
TUESDAY	Breakfast			
	Lunch			
	Dinner			
	Bedtime			
WEDNESDAY	Breakfast			
	Lunch			
	Dinner			
	Bedtime			
THURSDAY	Breakfast			
	Lunch			
	Dinner			
	Bedtime			
FRIDAY	Breakfast			
	Lunch			
	Dinner			
	Bedtime			
SATURDAY	Breakfast			
	Lunch			
	Dinner			
	Bedtime			
SUNDAY	Breakfast			
	Lunch			
	Dinner			
	Bedtime			

Weekly Blood Sugar Log

Week: _____ to _____

	Time	Before	After	Notes
MONDAY	Breakfast			
	Lunch			
	Dinner			
	Bedtime			
TUESDAY	Breakfast			
	Lunch			
	Dinner			
	Bedtime			
WEDNESDAY	Breakfast			
	Lunch			
	Dinner			
	Bedtime			
THURSDAY	Breakfast			
	Lunch			
	Dinner			
	Bedtime			
FRIDAY	Breakfast			
	Lunch			
	Dinner			
	Bedtime			
SATURDAY	Breakfast			
	Lunch			
	Dinner			
	Bedtime			
SUNDAY	Breakfast			
	Lunch			
	Dinner			
	Bedtime			

Weekly Blood Sugar Log

Week: _____ to _____

	Time	Before	After	Notes
MONDAY	Breakfast			
	Lunch			
	Dinner			
	Bedtime			
TUESDAY	Breakfast			
	Lunch			
	Dinner			
	Bedtime			
WEDNESDAY	Breakfast			
	Lunch			
	Dinner			
	Bedtime			
THURSDAY	Breakfast			
	Lunch			
	Dinner			
	Bedtime			
FRIDAY	Breakfast			
	Lunch			
	Dinner			
	Bedtime			
SATURDAY	Breakfast			
	Lunch			
	Dinner			
	Bedtime			
SUNDAY	Breakfast			
	Lunch			
	Dinner			
	Bedtime			

Weekly Blood Sugar Log

Week: _____ to _____

	Time	Before	After	Notes
MONDAY	Breakfast			
	Lunch			
	Dinner			
	Bedtime			
TUESDAY	Breakfast			
	Lunch			
	Dinner			
	Bedtime			
WEDNESDAY	Breakfast			
	Lunch			
	Dinner			
	Bedtime			
THURSDAY	Breakfast			
	Lunch			
	Dinner			
	Bedtime			
FRIDAY	Breakfast			
	Lunch			
	Dinner			
	Bedtime			
SATURDAY	Breakfast			
	Lunch			
	Dinner			
	Bedtime			
SUNDAY	Breakfast			
	Lunch			
	Dinner			
	Bedtime			

Weekly Blood Sugar Log

Week: _____ to _____

	Time	Before	After	Notes
MONDAY	Breakfast			
	Lunch			
	Dinner			
	Bedtime			
TUESDAY	Breakfast			
	Lunch			
	Dinner			
	Bedtime			
WEDNESDAY	Breakfast			
	Lunch			
	Dinner			
	Bedtime			
THURSDAY	Breakfast			
	Lunch			
	Dinner			
	Bedtime			
FRIDAY	Breakfast			
	Lunch			
	Dinner			
	Bedtime			
SATURDAY	Breakfast			
	Lunch			
	Dinner			
	Bedtime			
SUNDAY	Breakfast			
	Lunch			
	Dinner			
	Bedtime			

Weekly Blood Sugar Log

Week: _____ to _____

	Time	Before	After	Notes
MONDAY	Breakfast			
	Lunch			
	Dinner			
	Bedtime			
TUESDAY	Breakfast			
	Lunch			
	Dinner			
	Bedtime			
WEDNESDAY	Breakfast			
	Lunch			
	Dinner			
	Bedtime			
THURSDAY	Breakfast			
	Lunch			
	Dinner			
	Bedtime			
FRIDAY	Breakfast			
	Lunch			
	Dinner			
	Bedtime			
SATURDAY	Breakfast			
	Lunch			
	Dinner			
	Bedtime			
SUNDAY	Breakfast			
	Lunch			
	Dinner			
	Bedtime			

Weekly Blood Sugar Log

Week: _____ to _____

	Time	Before	After	Notes
MONDAY	Breakfast			
	Lunch			
	Dinner			
	Bedtime			
TUESDAY	Breakfast			
	Lunch			
	Dinner			
	Bedtime			
WEDNESDAY	Breakfast			
	Lunch			
	Dinner			
	Bedtime			
THURSDAY	Breakfast			
	Lunch			
	Dinner			
	Bedtime			
FRIDAY	Breakfast			
	Lunch			
	Dinner			
	Bedtime			
SATURDAY	Breakfast			
	Lunch			
	Dinner			
	Bedtime			
SUNDAY	Breakfast			
	Lunch			
	Dinner			
	Bedtime			

Weekly Blood Sugar Log

Week: _____ to _____

	Time	Before	After	Notes
MONDAY	Breakfast			
	Lunch			
	Dinner			
	Bedtime			
TUESDAY	Breakfast			
	Lunch			
	Dinner			
	Bedtime			
WEDNESDAY	Breakfast			
	Lunch			
	Dinner			
	Bedtime			
THURSDAY	Breakfast			
	Lunch			
	Dinner			
	Bedtime			
FRIDAY	Breakfast			
	Lunch			
	Dinner			
	Bedtime			
SATURDAY	Breakfast			
	Lunch			
	Dinner			
	Bedtime			
SUNDAY	Breakfast			
	Lunch			
	Dinner			
	Bedtime			

Weekly Blood Sugar Log

Week: _____ to _____

	Time	Before	After	Notes
MONDAY	Breakfast			
	Lunch			
	Dinner			
	Bedtime			
TUESDAY	Breakfast			
	Lunch			
	Dinner			
	Bedtime			
WEDNESDAY	Breakfast			
	Lunch			
	Dinner			
	Bedtime			
THURSDAY	Breakfast			
	Lunch			
	Dinner			
	Bedtime			
FRIDAY	Breakfast			
	Lunch			
	Dinner			
	Bedtime			
SATURDAY	Breakfast			
	Lunch			
	Dinner			
	Bedtime			
SUNDAY	Breakfast			
	Lunch			
	Dinner			
	Bedtime			

Weekly Blood Sugar Log

Week: _____ to _____

	Time	Before	After	Notes
MONDAY	Breakfast			
	Lunch			
	Dinner			
	Bedtime			
TUESDAY	Breakfast			
	Lunch			
	Dinner			
	Bedtime			
WEDNESDAY	Breakfast			
	Lunch			
	Dinner			
	Bedtime			
THURSDAY	Breakfast			
	Lunch			
	Dinner			
	Bedtime			
FRIDAY	Breakfast			
	Lunch			
	Dinner			
	Bedtime			
SATURDAY	Breakfast			
	Lunch			
	Dinner			
	Bedtime			
SUNDAY	Breakfast			
	Lunch			
	Dinner			
	Bedtime			

Weekly Blood Sugar Log

Week: _____ to _____

	Time	Before	After	Notes
MONDAY	Breakfast			
	Lunch			
	Dinner			
	Bedtime			
TUESDAY	Breakfast			
	Lunch			
	Dinner			
	Bedtime			
WEDNESDAY	Breakfast			
	Lunch			
	Dinner			
	Bedtime			
THURSDAY	Breakfast			
	Lunch			
	Dinner			
	Bedtime			
FRIDAY	Breakfast			
	Lunch			
	Dinner			
	Bedtime			
SATURDAY	Breakfast			
	Lunch			
	Dinner			
	Bedtime			
SUNDAY	Breakfast			
	Lunch			
	Dinner			
	Bedtime			

Weekly Blood Sugar Log

Week: _____ to _____

	Time	Before	After	Notes
MONDAY	Breakfast			
	Lunch			
	Dinner			
	Bedtime			
TUESDAY	Breakfast			
	Lunch			
	Dinner			
	Bedtime			
WEDNESDAY	Breakfast			
	Lunch			
	Dinner			
	Bedtime			
THURSDAY	Breakfast			
	Lunch			
	Dinner			
	Bedtime			
FRIDAY	Breakfast			
	Lunch			
	Dinner			
	Bedtime			
SATURDAY	Breakfast			
	Lunch			
	Dinner			
	Bedtime			
SUNDAY	Breakfast			
	Lunch			
	Dinner			
	Bedtime			

Weekly Blood Sugar Log

Week: _____ to _____

	Time	Before	After	Notes
MONDAY	Breakfast			
	Lunch			
	Dinner			
	Bedtime			
TUESDAY	Breakfast			
	Lunch			
	Dinner			
	Bedtime			
WEDNESDAY	Breakfast			
	Lunch			
	Dinner			
	Bedtime			
THURSDAY	Breakfast			
	Lunch			
	Dinner			
	Bedtime			
FRIDAY	Breakfast			
	Lunch			
	Dinner			
	Bedtime			
SATURDAY	Breakfast			
	Lunch			
	Dinner			
	Bedtime			
SUNDAY	Breakfast			
	Lunch			
	Dinner			
	Bedtime			

Weekly Blood Sugar Log

Week: _____ to _____

	Time	Before	After	Notes
MONDAY	Breakfast			
	Lunch			
	Dinner			
	Bedtime			
TUESDAY	Breakfast			
	Lunch			
	Dinner			
	Bedtime			
WEDNESDAY	Breakfast			
	Lunch			
	Dinner			
	Bedtime			
THURSDAY	Breakfast			
	Lunch			
	Dinner			
	Bedtime			
FRIDAY	Breakfast			
	Lunch			
	Dinner			
	Bedtime			
SATURDAY	Breakfast			
	Lunch			
	Dinner			
	Bedtime			
SUNDAY	Breakfast			
	Lunch			
	Dinner			
	Bedtime			

Weekly Blood Sugar Log

Week: _____ to _____

	Time	Before	After	Notes
MONDAY	Breakfast			
	Lunch			
	Dinner			
	Bedtime			
TUESDAY	Breakfast			
	Lunch			
	Dinner			
	Bedtime			
WEDNESDAY	Breakfast			
	Lunch			
	Dinner			
	Bedtime			
THURSDAY	Breakfast			
	Lunch			
	Dinner			
	Bedtime			
FRIDAY	Breakfast			
	Lunch			
	Dinner			
	Bedtime			
SATURDAY	Breakfast			
	Lunch			
	Dinner			
	Bedtime			
SUNDAY	Breakfast			
	Lunch			
	Dinner			
	Bedtime			

Weekly Blood Sugar Log

Week: _____ to _____

	Time	Before	After	Notes
MONDAY	Breakfast			
	Lunch			
	Dinner			
	Bedtime			
TUESDAY	Breakfast			
	Lunch			
	Dinner			
	Bedtime			
WEDNESDAY	Breakfast			
	Lunch			
	Dinner			
	Bedtime			
THURSDAY	Breakfast			
	Lunch			
	Dinner			
	Bedtime			
FRIDAY	Breakfast			
	Lunch			
	Dinner			
	Bedtime			
SATURDAY	Breakfast			
	Lunch			
	Dinner			
	Bedtime			
SUNDAY	Breakfast			
	Lunch			
	Dinner			
	Bedtime			

Weekly Blood Sugar Log

Week: _____ to _____

	Time	Before	After	Notes
MONDAY	Breakfast			
	Lunch			
	Dinner			
	Bedtime			
TUESDAY	Breakfast			
	Lunch			
	Dinner			
	Bedtime			
WEDNESDAY	Breakfast			
	Lunch			
	Dinner			
	Bedtime			
THURSDAY	Breakfast			
	Lunch			
	Dinner			
	Bedtime			
FRIDAY	Breakfast			
	Lunch			
	Dinner			
	Bedtime			
SATURDAY	Breakfast			
	Lunch			
	Dinner			
	Bedtime			
SUNDAY	Breakfast			
	Lunch			
	Dinner			
	Bedtime			

Weekly Blood Sugar Log

Week: _____ to _____

	Time	Before	After	Notes
MONDAY	Breakfast			
	Lunch			
	Dinner			
	Bedtime			
TUESDAY	Breakfast			
	Lunch			
	Dinner			
	Bedtime			
WEDNESDAY	Breakfast			
	Lunch			
	Dinner			
	Bedtime			
THURSDAY	Breakfast			
	Lunch			
	Dinner			
	Bedtime			
FRIDAY	Breakfast			
	Lunch			
	Dinner			
	Bedtime			
SATURDAY	Breakfast			
	Lunch			
	Dinner			
	Bedtime			
SUNDAY	Breakfast			
	Lunch			
	Dinner			
	Bedtime			

Weekly Blood Sugar Log

Week: _____ to _____

	Time	Before	After	Notes
MONDAY	Breakfast			
	Lunch			
	Dinner			
	Bedtime			
TUESDAY	Breakfast			
	Lunch			
	Dinner			
	Bedtime			
WEDNESDAY	Breakfast			
	Lunch			
	Dinner			
	Bedtime			
THURSDAY	Breakfast			
	Lunch			
	Dinner			
	Bedtime			
FRIDAY	Breakfast			
	Lunch			
	Dinner			
	Bedtime			
SATURDAY	Breakfast			
	Lunch			
	Dinner			
	Bedtime			
SUNDAY	Breakfast			
	Lunch			
	Dinner			
	Bedtime			

Weekly Blood Sugar Log

Week: _____ to _____

	Time	Before	After	Notes
MONDAY	Breakfast			
	Lunch			
	Dinner			
	Bedtime			
TUESDAY	Breakfast			
	Lunch			
	Dinner			
	Bedtime			
WEDNESDAY	Breakfast			
	Lunch			
	Dinner			
	Bedtime			
THURSDAY	Breakfast			
	Lunch			
	Dinner			
	Bedtime			
FRIDAY	Breakfast			
	Lunch			
	Dinner			
	Bedtime			
SATURDAY	Breakfast			
	Lunch			
	Dinner			
	Bedtime			
SUNDAY	Breakfast			
	Lunch			
	Dinner			
	Bedtime			

Weekly Blood Sugar Log

Week: _____ to _____

	Time	Before	After	Notes
MONDAY	Breakfast			
	Lunch			
	Dinner			
	Bedtime			
TUESDAY	Breakfast			
	Lunch			
	Dinner			
	Bedtime			
WEDNESDAY	Breakfast			
	Lunch			
	Dinner			
	Bedtime			
THURSDAY	Breakfast			
	Lunch			
	Dinner			
	Bedtime			
FRIDAY	Breakfast			
	Lunch			
	Dinner			
	Bedtime			
SATURDAY	Breakfast			
	Lunch			
	Dinner			
	Bedtime			
SUNDAY	Breakfast			
	Lunch			
	Dinner			
	Bedtime			

Weekly Blood Sugar Log

Week: _____ to _____

	Time	Before	After	Notes
MONDAY	Breakfast			
	Lunch			
	Dinner			
	Bedtime			
TUESDAY	Breakfast			
	Lunch			
	Dinner			
	Bedtime			
WEDNESDAY	Breakfast			
	Lunch			
	Dinner			
	Bedtime			
THURSDAY	Breakfast			
	Lunch			
	Dinner			
	Bedtime			
FRIDAY	Breakfast			
	Lunch			
	Dinner			
	Bedtime			
SATURDAY	Breakfast			
	Lunch			
	Dinner			
	Bedtime			
SUNDAY	Breakfast			
	Lunch			
	Dinner			
	Bedtime			

Weekly Blood Sugar Log

Week: _____ to _____

	Time	Before	After	Notes
MONDAY	Breakfast			
	Lunch			
	Dinner			
	Bedtime			
TUESDAY	Breakfast			
	Lunch			
	Dinner			
	Bedtime			
WEDNESDAY	Breakfast			
	Lunch			
	Dinner			
	Bedtime			
THURSDAY	Breakfast			
	Lunch			
	Dinner			
	Bedtime			
FRIDAY	Breakfast			
	Lunch			
	Dinner			
	Bedtime			
SATURDAY	Breakfast			
	Lunch			
	Dinner			
	Bedtime			
SUNDAY	Breakfast			
	Lunch			
	Dinner			
	Bedtime			

Weekly Blood Sugar Log

Week: _____ to _____

	Time	Before	After	Notes
MONDAY	Breakfast			
	Lunch			
	Dinner			
	Bedtime			
TUESDAY	Breakfast			
	Lunch			
	Dinner			
	Bedtime			
WEDNESDAY	Breakfast			
	Lunch			
	Dinner			
	Bedtime			
THURSDAY	Breakfast			
	Lunch			
	Dinner			
	Bedtime			
FRIDAY	Breakfast			
	Lunch			
	Dinner			
	Bedtime			
SATURDAY	Breakfast			
	Lunch			
	Dinner			
	Bedtime			
SUNDAY	Breakfast			
	Lunch			
	Dinner			
	Bedtime			

Weekly Blood Sugar Log

Week: _____ to _____

	Time	Before	After	Notes
MONDAY	Breakfast			
	Lunch			
	Dinner			
	Bedtime			
TUESDAY	Breakfast			
	Lunch			
	Dinner			
	Bedtime			
WEDNESDAY	Breakfast			
	Lunch			
	Dinner			
	Bedtime			
THURSDAY	Breakfast			
	Lunch			
	Dinner			
	Bedtime			
FRIDAY	Breakfast			
	Lunch			
	Dinner			
	Bedtime			
SATURDAY	Breakfast			
	Lunch			
	Dinner			
	Bedtime			
SUNDAY	Breakfast			
	Lunch			
	Dinner			
	Bedtime			

Weekly Blood Sugar Log

Week: _____ to _____

	Time	Before	After	Notes
MONDAY	Breakfast			
	Lunch			
	Dinner			
	Bedtime			
TUESDAY	Breakfast			
	Lunch			
	Dinner			
	Bedtime			
WEDNESDAY	Breakfast			
	Lunch			
	Dinner			
	Bedtime			
THURSDAY	Breakfast			
	Lunch			
	Dinner			
	Bedtime			
FRIDAY	Breakfast			
	Lunch			
	Dinner			
	Bedtime			
SATURDAY	Breakfast			
	Lunch			
	Dinner			
	Bedtime			
SUNDAY	Breakfast			
	Lunch			
	Dinner			
	Bedtime			

Weekly Blood Sugar Log

Week: _____ to _____

	Time	Before	After	Notes
MONDAY	Breakfast			
	Lunch			
	Dinner			
	Bedtime			
TUESDAY	Breakfast			
	Lunch			
	Dinner			
	Bedtime			
WEDNESDAY	Breakfast			
	Lunch			
	Dinner			
	Bedtime			
THURSDAY	Breakfast			
	Lunch			
	Dinner			
	Bedtime			
FRIDAY	Breakfast			
	Lunch			
	Dinner			
	Bedtime			
SATURDAY	Breakfast			
	Lunch			
	Dinner			
	Bedtime			
SUNDAY	Breakfast			
	Lunch			
	Dinner			
	Bedtime			

Weekly Blood Sugar Log

Week: _____ to _____

	Time	Before	After	Notes
MONDAY	Breakfast			
	Lunch			
	Dinner			
	Bedtime			
TUESDAY	Breakfast			
	Lunch			
	Dinner			
	Bedtime			
WEDNESDAY	Breakfast			
	Lunch			
	Dinner			
	Bedtime			
THURSDAY	Breakfast			
	Lunch			
	Dinner			
	Bedtime			
FRIDAY	Breakfast			
	Lunch			
	Dinner			
	Bedtime			
SATURDAY	Breakfast			
	Lunch			
	Dinner			
	Bedtime			
SUNDAY	Breakfast			
	Lunch			
	Dinner			
	Bedtime			

Weekly Blood Sugar Log

Week: _____ to _____

	Time	Before	After	Notes
MONDAY	Breakfast			
	Lunch			
	Dinner			
	Bedtime			
TUESDAY	Breakfast			
	Lunch			
	Dinner			
	Bedtime			
WEDNESDAY	Breakfast			
	Lunch			
	Dinner			
	Bedtime			
THURSDAY	Breakfast			
	Lunch			
	Dinner			
	Bedtime			
FRIDAY	Breakfast			
	Lunch			
	Dinner			
	Bedtime			
SATURDAY	Breakfast			
	Lunch			
	Dinner			
	Bedtime			
SUNDAY	Breakfast			
	Lunch			
	Dinner			
	Bedtime			

Weekly Blood Sugar Log

Week: _____ to _____

	Time	Before	After	Notes
MONDAY	Breakfast			
	Lunch			
	Dinner			
	Bedtime			
TUESDAY	Breakfast			
	Lunch			
	Dinner			
	Bedtime			
WEDNESDAY	Breakfast			
	Lunch			
	Dinner			
	Bedtime			
THURSDAY	Breakfast			
	Lunch			
	Dinner			
	Bedtime			
FRIDAY	Breakfast			
	Lunch			
	Dinner			
	Bedtime			
SATURDAY	Breakfast			
	Lunch			
	Dinner			
	Bedtime			
SUNDAY	Breakfast			
	Lunch			
	Dinner			
	Bedtime			

Weekly Blood Sugar Log

Week: _____ to _____

	Time	Before	After	Notes
MONDAY	Breakfast			
	Lunch			
	Dinner			
	Bedtime			
TUESDAY	Breakfast			
	Lunch			
	Dinner			
	Bedtime			
WEDNESDAY	Breakfast			
	Lunch			
	Dinner			
	Bedtime			
THURSDAY	Breakfast			
	Lunch			
	Dinner			
	Bedtime			
FRIDAY	Breakfast			
	Lunch			
	Dinner			
	Bedtime			
SATURDAY	Breakfast			
	Lunch			
	Dinner			
	Bedtime			
SUNDAY	Breakfast			
	Lunch			
	Dinner			
	Bedtime			

Weekly Blood Sugar Log

Week: _____ to _____

	Time	Before	After	Notes
MONDAY	Breakfast			
	Lunch			
	Dinner			
	Bedtime			
TUESDAY	Breakfast			
	Lunch			
	Dinner			
	Bedtime			
WEDNESDAY	Breakfast			
	Lunch			
	Dinner			
	Bedtime			
THURSDAY	Breakfast			
	Lunch			
	Dinner			
	Bedtime			
FRIDAY	Breakfast			
	Lunch			
	Dinner			
	Bedtime			
SATURDAY	Breakfast			
	Lunch			
	Dinner			
	Bedtime			
SUNDAY	Breakfast			
	Lunch			
	Dinner			
	Bedtime			

Weekly Blood Sugar Log

Week: _____ to _____

	Time	Before	After	Notes
MONDAY	Breakfast			
	Lunch			
	Dinner			
	Bedtime			
TUESDAY	Breakfast			
	Lunch			
	Dinner			
	Bedtime			
WEDNESDAY	Breakfast			
	Lunch			
	Dinner			
	Bedtime			
THURSDAY	Breakfast			
	Lunch			
	Dinner			
	Bedtime			
FRIDAY	Breakfast			
	Lunch			
	Dinner			
	Bedtime			
SATURDAY	Breakfast			
	Lunch			
	Dinner			
	Bedtime			
SUNDAY	Breakfast			
	Lunch			
	Dinner			
	Bedtime			

Weekly Blood Sugar Log

Week: _____ to _____

	Time	Before	After	Notes
MONDAY	Breakfast			
	Lunch			
	Dinner			
	Bedtime			
TUESDAY	Breakfast			
	Lunch			
	Dinner			
	Bedtime			
WEDNESDAY	Breakfast			
	Lunch			
	Dinner			
	Bedtime			
THURSDAY	Breakfast			
	Lunch			
	Dinner			
	Bedtime			
FRIDAY	Breakfast			
	Lunch			
	Dinner			
	Bedtime			
SATURDAY	Breakfast			
	Lunch			
	Dinner			
	Bedtime			
SUNDAY	Breakfast			
	Lunch			
	Dinner			
	Bedtime			

Weekly Blood Sugar Log

Week: _____ to _____

	Time	Before	After	Notes
MONDAY	Breakfast			
	Lunch			
	Dinner			
	Bedtime			
TUESDAY	Breakfast			
	Lunch			
	Dinner			
	Bedtime			
WEDNESDAY	Breakfast			
	Lunch			
	Dinner			
	Bedtime			
THURSDAY	Breakfast			
	Lunch			
	Dinner			
	Bedtime			
FRIDAY	Breakfast			
	Lunch			
	Dinner			
	Bedtime			
SATURDAY	Breakfast			
	Lunch			
	Dinner			
	Bedtime			
SUNDAY	Breakfast			
	Lunch			
	Dinner			
	Bedtime			

Weekly Blood Sugar Log

Week: _____ to _____

	Time	Before	After	Notes
MONDAY	Breakfast			
	Lunch			
	Dinner			
	Bedtime			
TUESDAY	Breakfast			
	Lunch			
	Dinner			
	Bedtime			
WEDNESDAY	Breakfast			
	Lunch			
	Dinner			
	Bedtime			
THURSDAY	Breakfast			
	Lunch			
	Dinner			
	Bedtime			
FRIDAY	Breakfast			
	Lunch			
	Dinner			
	Bedtime			
SATURDAY	Breakfast			
	Lunch			
	Dinner			
	Bedtime			
SUNDAY	Breakfast			
	Lunch			
	Dinner			
	Bedtime			

Weekly Blood Sugar Log

Week: _____ to _____

	Time	Before	After	Notes
MONDAY	Breakfast			
	Lunch			
	Dinner			
	Bedtime			
TUESDAY	Breakfast			
	Lunch			
	Dinner			
	Bedtime			
WEDNESDAY	Breakfast			
	Lunch			
	Dinner			
	Bedtime			
THURSDAY	Breakfast			
	Lunch			
	Dinner			
	Bedtime			
FRIDAY	Breakfast			
	Lunch			
	Dinner			
	Bedtime			
SATURDAY	Breakfast			
	Lunch			
	Dinner			
	Bedtime			
SUNDAY	Breakfast			
	Lunch			
	Dinner			
	Bedtime			

Weekly Blood Sugar Log

Week: _____ to _____

	Time	Before	After	Notes
MONDAY	Breakfast			
	Lunch			
	Dinner			
	Bedtime			
TUESDAY	Breakfast			
	Lunch			
	Dinner			
	Bedtime			
WEDNESDAY	Breakfast			
	Lunch			
	Dinner			
	Bedtime			
THURSDAY	Breakfast			
	Lunch			
	Dinner			
	Bedtime			
FRIDAY	Breakfast			
	Lunch			
	Dinner			
	Bedtime			
SATURDAY	Breakfast			
	Lunch			
	Dinner			
	Bedtime			
SUNDAY	Breakfast			
	Lunch			
	Dinner			
	Bedtime			

Weekly Blood Sugar Log

Week: _____ to _____

	Time	Before	After	Notes
MONDAY	Breakfast			
	Lunch			
	Dinner			
	Bedtime			
TUESDAY	Breakfast			
	Lunch			
	Dinner			
	Bedtime			
WEDNESDAY	Breakfast			
	Lunch			
	Dinner			
	Bedtime			
THURSDAY	Breakfast			
	Lunch			
	Dinner			
	Bedtime			
FRIDAY	Breakfast			
	Lunch			
	Dinner			
	Bedtime			
SATURDAY	Breakfast			
	Lunch			
	Dinner			
	Bedtime			
SUNDAY	Breakfast			
	Lunch			
	Dinner			
	Bedtime			

Weekly Blood Sugar Log

Week: _____ to _____

	Time	Before	After	Notes
MONDAY	Breakfast			
	Lunch			
	Dinner			
	Bedtime			
TUESDAY	Breakfast			
	Lunch			
	Dinner			
	Bedtime			
WEDNESDAY	Breakfast			
	Lunch			
	Dinner			
	Bedtime			
THURSDAY	Breakfast			
	Lunch			
	Dinner			
	Bedtime			
FRIDAY	Breakfast			
	Lunch			
	Dinner			
	Bedtime			
SATURDAY	Breakfast			
	Lunch			
	Dinner			
	Bedtime			
SUNDAY	Breakfast			
	Lunch			
	Dinner			
	Bedtime			

Weekly Blood Sugar Log

Week: _____ to _____

	Time	Before	After	Notes
MONDAY	Breakfast			
	Lunch			
	Dinner			
	Bedtime			
TUESDAY	Breakfast			
	Lunch			
	Dinner			
	Bedtime			
WEDNESDAY	Breakfast			
	Lunch			
	Dinner			
	Bedtime			
THURSDAY	Breakfast			
	Lunch			
	Dinner			
	Bedtime			
FRIDAY	Breakfast			
	Lunch			
	Dinner			
	Bedtime			
SATURDAY	Breakfast			
	Lunch			
	Dinner			
	Bedtime			
SUNDAY	Breakfast			
	Lunch			
	Dinner			
	Bedtime			

Weekly Blood Sugar Log

Week: _____ to _____

	Time	Before	After	Notes
MONDAY	Breakfast			
	Lunch			
	Dinner			
	Bedtime			
TUESDAY	Breakfast			
	Lunch			
	Dinner			
	Bedtime			
WEDNESDAY	Breakfast			
	Lunch			
	Dinner			
	Bedtime			
THURSDAY	Breakfast			
	Lunch			
	Dinner			
	Bedtime			
FRIDAY	Breakfast			
	Lunch			
	Dinner			
	Bedtime			
SATURDAY	Breakfast			
	Lunch			
	Dinner			
	Bedtime			
SUNDAY	Breakfast			
	Lunch			
	Dinner			
	Bedtime			

Weekly Blood Sugar Log

Week: _____ to _____

	Time	Before	After	Notes
MONDAY	Breakfast			
	Lunch			
	Dinner			
	Bedtime			
TUESDAY	Breakfast			
	Lunch			
	Dinner			
	Bedtime			
WEDNESDAY	Breakfast			
	Lunch			
	Dinner			
	Bedtime			
THURSDAY	Breakfast			
	Lunch			
	Dinner			
	Bedtime			
FRIDAY	Breakfast			
	Lunch			
	Dinner			
	Bedtime			
SATURDAY	Breakfast			
	Lunch			
	Dinner			
	Bedtime			
SUNDAY	Breakfast			
	Lunch			
	Dinner			
	Bedtime			

Weekly Blood Sugar Log

Week: _____ to _____

	Time	Before	After	Notes
MONDAY	Breakfast			
	Lunch			
	Dinner			
	Bedtime			
TUESDAY	Breakfast			
	Lunch			
	Dinner			
	Bedtime			
WEDNESDAY	Breakfast			
	Lunch			
	Dinner			
	Bedtime			
THURSDAY	Breakfast			
	Lunch			
	Dinner			
	Bedtime			
FRIDAY	Breakfast			
	Lunch			
	Dinner			
	Bedtime			
SATURDAY	Breakfast			
	Lunch			
	Dinner			
	Bedtime			
SUNDAY	Breakfast			
	Lunch			
	Dinner			
	Bedtime			

Weekly Blood Sugar Log

Week: _____ to _____

	Time	Before	After	Notes
MONDAY	Breakfast			
	Lunch			
	Dinner			
	Bedtime			
TUESDAY	Breakfast			
	Lunch			
	Dinner			
	Bedtime			
WEDNESDAY	Breakfast			
	Lunch			
	Dinner			
	Bedtime			
THURSDAY	Breakfast			
	Lunch			
	Dinner			
	Bedtime			
FRIDAY	Breakfast			
	Lunch			
	Dinner			
	Bedtime			
SATURDAY	Breakfast			
	Lunch			
	Dinner			
	Bedtime			
SUNDAY	Breakfast			
	Lunch			
	Dinner			
	Bedtime			

Weekly Blood Sugar Log

Week: _____ to _____

	Time	Before	After	Notes
MONDAY	Breakfast			
	Lunch			
	Dinner			
	Bedtime			
TUESDAY	Breakfast			
	Lunch			
	Dinner			
	Bedtime			
WEDNESDAY	Breakfast			
	Lunch			
	Dinner			
	Bedtime			
THURSDAY	Breakfast			
	Lunch			
	Dinner			
	Bedtime			
FRIDAY	Breakfast			
	Lunch			
	Dinner			
	Bedtime			
SATURDAY	Breakfast			
	Lunch			
	Dinner			
	Bedtime			
SUNDAY	Breakfast			
	Lunch			
	Dinner			
	Bedtime			

Weekly Blood Sugar Log

Week: _____ to _____

	Time	Before	After	Notes
MONDAY	Breakfast			
	Lunch			
	Dinner			
	Bedtime			
TUESDAY	Breakfast			
	Lunch			
	Dinner			
	Bedtime			
WEDNESDAY	Breakfast			
	Lunch			
	Dinner			
	Bedtime			
THURSDAY	Breakfast			
	Lunch			
	Dinner			
	Bedtime			
FRIDAY	Breakfast			
	Lunch			
	Dinner			
	Bedtime			
SATURDAY	Breakfast			
	Lunch			
	Dinner			
	Bedtime			
SUNDAY	Breakfast			
	Lunch			
	Dinner			
	Bedtime			

Weekly Blood Sugar Log

Week: _____ to _____

	Time	Before	After	Notes
MONDAY	Breakfast			
	Lunch			
	Dinner			
	Bedtime			
TUESDAY	Breakfast			
	Lunch			
	Dinner			
	Bedtime			
WEDNESDAY	Breakfast			
	Lunch			
	Dinner			
	Bedtime			
THURSDAY	Breakfast			
	Lunch			
	Dinner			
	Bedtime			
FRIDAY	Breakfast			
	Lunch			
	Dinner			
	Bedtime			
SATURDAY	Breakfast			
	Lunch			
	Dinner			
	Bedtime			
SUNDAY	Breakfast			
	Lunch			
	Dinner			
	Bedtime			

Weekly Blood Sugar Log

Week: _____ to _____

	Time	Before	After	Notes
MONDAY	Breakfast			
	Lunch			
	Dinner			
	Bedtime			
TUESDAY	Breakfast			
	Lunch			
	Dinner			
	Bedtime			
WEDNESDAY	Breakfast			
	Lunch			
	Dinner			
	Bedtime			
THURSDAY	Breakfast			
	Lunch			
	Dinner			
	Bedtime			
FRIDAY	Breakfast			
	Lunch			
	Dinner			
	Bedtime			
SATURDAY	Breakfast			
	Lunch			
	Dinner			
	Bedtime			
SUNDAY	Breakfast			
	Lunch			
	Dinner			
	Bedtime			

Weekly Blood Sugar Log

Week: _____ to _____

	Time	Before	After	Notes
MONDAY	Breakfast			
	Lunch			
	Dinner			
	Bedtime			
TUESDAY	Breakfast			
	Lunch			
	Dinner			
	Bedtime			
WEDNESDAY	Breakfast			
	Lunch			
	Dinner			
	Bedtime			
THURSDAY	Breakfast			
	Lunch			
	Dinner			
	Bedtime			
FRIDAY	Breakfast			
	Lunch			
	Dinner			
	Bedtime			
SATURDAY	Breakfast			
	Lunch			
	Dinner			
	Bedtime			
SUNDAY	Breakfast			
	Lunch			
	Dinner			
	Bedtime			

Weekly Blood Sugar Log

Week: _____ to _____

	Time	Before	After	Notes
MONDAY	Breakfast			
	Lunch			
	Dinner			
	Bedtime			
TUESDAY	Breakfast			
	Lunch			
	Dinner			
	Bedtime			
WEDNESDAY	Breakfast			
	Lunch			
	Dinner			
	Bedtime			
THURSDAY	Breakfast			
	Lunch			
	Dinner			
	Bedtime			
FRIDAY	Breakfast			
	Lunch			
	Dinner			
	Bedtime			
SATURDAY	Breakfast			
	Lunch			
	Dinner			
	Bedtime			
SUNDAY	Breakfast			
	Lunch			
	Dinner			
	Bedtime			

Weekly Blood Sugar Log

Week: _____ to _____

	Time	Before	After	Notes
MONDAY	Breakfast			
	Lunch			
	Dinner			
	Bedtime			
TUESDAY	Breakfast			
	Lunch			
	Dinner			
	Bedtime			
WEDNESDAY	Breakfast			
	Lunch			
	Dinner			
	Bedtime			
THURSDAY	Breakfast			
	Lunch			
	Dinner			
	Bedtime			
FRIDAY	Breakfast			
	Lunch			
	Dinner			
	Bedtime			
SATURDAY	Breakfast			
	Lunch			
	Dinner			
	Bedtime			
SUNDAY	Breakfast			
	Lunch			
	Dinner			
	Bedtime			

Weekly Blood Sugar Log

Week: _____ to _____

	Time	Before	After	Notes
MONDAY	Breakfast			
	Lunch			
	Dinner			
	Bedtime			
TUESDAY	Breakfast			
	Lunch			
	Dinner			
	Bedtime			
WEDNESDAY	Breakfast			
	Lunch			
	Dinner			
	Bedtime			
THURSDAY	Breakfast			
	Lunch			
	Dinner			
	Bedtime			
FRIDAY	Breakfast			
	Lunch			
	Dinner			
	Bedtime			
SATURDAY	Breakfast			
	Lunch			
	Dinner			
	Bedtime			
SUNDAY	Breakfast			
	Lunch			
	Dinner			
	Bedtime			

Weekly Blood Sugar Log

Week: _____ to _____

	Time	Before	After	Notes
MONDAY	Breakfast			
	Lunch			
	Dinner			
	Bedtime			
TUESDAY	Breakfast			
	Lunch			
	Dinner			
	Bedtime			
WEDNESDAY	Breakfast			
	Lunch			
	Dinner			
	Bedtime			
THURSDAY	Breakfast			
	Lunch			
	Dinner			
	Bedtime			
FRIDAY	Breakfast			
	Lunch			
	Dinner			
	Bedtime			
SATURDAY	Breakfast			
	Lunch			
	Dinner			
	Bedtime			
SUNDAY	Breakfast			
	Lunch			
	Dinner			
	Bedtime			

Weekly Blood Sugar Log

Week: _____ to _____

	Time	Before	After	Notes
MONDAY	Breakfast			
	Lunch			
	Dinner			
	Bedtime			
TUESDAY	Breakfast			
	Lunch			
	Dinner			
	Bedtime			
WEDNESDAY	Breakfast			
	Lunch			
	Dinner			
	Bedtime			
THURSDAY	Breakfast			
	Lunch			
	Dinner			
	Bedtime			
FRIDAY	Breakfast			
	Lunch			
	Dinner			
	Bedtime			
SATURDAY	Breakfast			
	Lunch			
	Dinner			
	Bedtime			
SUNDAY	Breakfast			
	Lunch			
	Dinner			
	Bedtime			

Weekly Blood Sugar Log

Week: _____ to _____

	Time	Before	After	Notes
MONDAY	Breakfast			
	Lunch			
	Dinner			
	Bedtime			
TUESDAY	Breakfast			
	Lunch			
	Dinner			
	Bedtime			
WEDNESDAY	Breakfast			
	Lunch			
	Dinner			
	Bedtime			
THURSDAY	Breakfast			
	Lunch			
	Dinner			
	Bedtime			
FRIDAY	Breakfast			
	Lunch			
	Dinner			
	Bedtime			
SATURDAY	Breakfast			
	Lunch			
	Dinner			
	Bedtime			
SUNDAY	Breakfast			
	Lunch			
	Dinner			
	Bedtime			

Weekly Blood Sugar Log

Week: _____ to _____

	Time	Before	After	Notes
MONDAY	Breakfast			
	Lunch			
	Dinner			
	Bedtime			
TUESDAY	Breakfast			
	Lunch			
	Dinner			
	Bedtime			
WEDNESDAY	Breakfast			
	Lunch			
	Dinner			
	Bedtime			
THURSDAY	Breakfast			
	Lunch			
	Dinner			
	Bedtime			
FRIDAY	Breakfast			
	Lunch			
	Dinner			
	Bedtime			
SATURDAY	Breakfast			
	Lunch			
	Dinner			
	Bedtime			
SUNDAY	Breakfast			
	Lunch			
	Dinner			
	Bedtime			

Weekly Blood Sugar Log

Week: _____ to _____

	Time	Before	After	Notes
MONDAY	Breakfast			
	Lunch			
	Dinner			
	Bedtime			
TUESDAY	Breakfast			
	Lunch			
	Dinner			
	Bedtime			
WEDNESDAY	Breakfast			
	Lunch			
	Dinner			
	Bedtime			
THURSDAY	Breakfast			
	Lunch			
	Dinner			
	Bedtime			
FRIDAY	Breakfast			
	Lunch			
	Dinner			
	Bedtime			
SATURDAY	Breakfast			
	Lunch			
	Dinner			
	Bedtime			
SUNDAY	Breakfast			
	Lunch			
	Dinner			
	Bedtime			

Weekly Blood Sugar Log

Week: _____ to _____

	Time	Before	After	Notes
MONDAY	Breakfast			
	Lunch			
	Dinner			
	Bedtime			
TUESDAY	Breakfast			
	Lunch			
	Dinner			
	Bedtime			
WEDNESDAY	Breakfast			
	Lunch			
	Dinner			
	Bedtime			
THURSDAY	Breakfast			
	Lunch			
	Dinner			
	Bedtime			
FRIDAY	Breakfast			
	Lunch			
	Dinner			
	Bedtime			
SATURDAY	Breakfast			
	Lunch			
	Dinner			
	Bedtime			
SUNDAY	Breakfast			
	Lunch			
	Dinner			
	Bedtime			

Notes:

Notes:

Made in the USA
Monee, IL
06 January 2023

24653453R00061